The Cookbook for a Compassionate Nurse

An important recipe for nursing.

LUZMARIE HAWKINS

Copyright © 2019 Luzmarie Hawkins

All rights reserved.

ISBN-13: 9781798571354

DEDICATION

I dedicate this book to my loving husband who has stood by my side, supporting me and sacrificing his wants and needs so that I could go back to school to achieve my goals. To my mother, who taught me the meaning of compassion and love. To my beautiful children, who motivate me to be the best I can be.

& To the King of my heart, my heavenly Father.

CONTENTS

	INTRO	vi
1	Nursing	1
2	Competence	5
3	Understanding	15
4	Attention to Detail	21
5	Endurance	25
6	Honesty	28
7	No Judgement	33
8	Compassion	37
	About the Author	47

Nutrition Facts

Servings Size   1 Compassionate Nurse*

Amount Per Serving

P.R.N. (As Needed)

	% Daily Value *
Competence	1000%
Understanding	500%
Attention to Detail	900%
Endurance	700%
Honesty	2000%
Judgemental	0%
Compassion	Infinite

---

*Not a Significant Source of Value Received.
**Percent Daily Values are Based on Your Individual Diet.

INTRO

My desire to enter the health care field began when I was a little girl. In kindergarten, my favorite part of the day was play time where we all dressed up as anything we wanted to be. I found myself always running to the white lab coat and being the first one to grab the medical supplies. Already at a young age, my desire was to save lives. I wanted to help take care of others and heal them. At 6 years old, I knew right away that it was my duty to serve others. There was a feeling I got in my stomach, like butterflies, whenever my "first patient" of the day would come to my pretend office for their check-up. Those days came and went faster than I can remember and soon, I had desires for many other things.

I wanted to be a singer, an artist, a cosmetologist, a teacher, you name it! I think it's normal for young adults to change their mind on their career path a million times before they finally settle (or not settle) on one. I considered myself in the "or not settle" category because I tapped into more of my creative side as I got older. No matter what life threw my way, though, I never let go of my dream of becoming a doctor.

I watched my mother constantly occupy herself with arts and crafts and I remember how happy it made her. I shared those moments with my mother. I wanted to experience that happiness by joining her in all things artistic and crafty. I soon learned how to do nails, specializing in acrylics. I even learned how to use ia sewing machine to make my daughter her own clothes and created a custom car seat for her too. I then began creating these beautifully sculpted custom cakes that eventually turned into a home business. While all these awesome talents branched off from me, I still pursued a career in health care and went back to school for nursing.

My journey through nursing has been a rough one. I battled with feelings of confusion, disappointment, and depression. It has been a journey that I can pair with the word bittersweet. Among all the beautiful rewarding successes, there have been plenty of moments that brought me to some low points. Baking and decorating cakes have been my stress-relievers at times when I felt overwhelmed in nursing school. Once I began working as a nurse, creating edible artwork was my getaway. Now, don't get to thinking that being a cake artist wasn't stressful because it sure was at many times. But no matter how crazy it got, no matter how many orders piled up, no matter how many days I went without eating and nights without sleeping, the end results always brought me joy.

So, now that I have explained a little bit about my background, I feel that I can tell you why I chose to write a book about nursing in the format of a cookbook. I realized that whatever I did in life, in my case being a cake artist and nurse, they all had one common denominator: compassion. The qualities of a compassionate person are the strongest pieces of the solid foundation for whatever it is you decide to do in your life. Just as you must have the correct recipe to create a delicious meal or dessert, you must have the correct recipe to be successful in life.

In nursing school, the instructors teach you about all the fundamentals and clinical work it takes to be successful, but they are missing one important part. Teaching future nurses the first and most important quality is crucial in today's world, and I believe it's compassion. Nurses should truly understand and be able to display compassion within their work. By incorporating it in your career and life, it can truly change how you care for others and yourselves. We all want the same things in life: love, attention, happiness, the feeling of importance, and success. Every single person on this Earth wants to feel joy. If we could focus on spreading compassion despite how we feel at the moment, I believe it could make a world of a difference. No one ever feels horrible after sharing a kind word or a smile. I hope my book can shine an everlasting light that guides you on the path of love in this dark world.

CHAPTER 1

Nursing

    It all begins with someone caring. Caring to make someone well again, to help them heal, to prevent illness, to see someone overcome obstacles in their health, and to be joyful once again. Nurses not only change lives, but they save lives. The nurturing touch that they give and the compassion that they impart into a patient does something more incredible than medicine could ever do. It heals the heart and comforts the soul. It brings a love and peace that washes away fears and anxieties. Compassion allows trust to become established and resting to take place.

    Imagine a flower and how it grows. The seed must be planted in the right soil, in the right environment. It must then receive the right amount of water and sun to encourage growth. Weeds will grow all around it as it begins to bloom. The weeds must be removed carefully to not damage the growing flower. The beauty and the multitude of varieties of flowers that grow together under the same soil is truly an amazing wonder of God. From where a tree grows, a bed of beautiful flowers may grow as well. There is no discrimination on which one gets more water and care, no matter how big or how little the plant may be. They thrive and grow among one another, creating beautiful landscapes and scenery. They all have their seasons to flourish and seasons to rest. The tree, the flower, and the seed are all cared for during every season.

We are all individually chosen and carefully created with greater detail and care than the birds of the sky and the plants of the earth. We do, however, have a lot of things in common. We must be planted and nurtured in the right environment, with all the right nourishments needed to grow. We must be fed with positive and uplifting things and filled with the right knowledge to become successful through life's challenges. As time goes on, we also have weeds that grow around us. We must be aware of them as they can hinder our growth. As hard as it may be, we must cut the weeds out of our life – the people, habits, and unhealthy life choices. In the end, we grow and we bloom. Some of us become strong, tall trees, and some of us become small, fragile, gorgeous flowers in the garden. Nursing is very comparable to the beauty and life in nature. How could you expect a person to become a successful healing caregiver without giving them the proper education and support for their own personal health and wellness journey?

I will tell you right now from my experience, not only in LPN school but in RN school as well, finishing a nursing program was one of the most difficult journeys I have been on. Nursing school is NOT EASY, and it can definitely wear you down. It is tough on its own, let along having little to no support through it. You will focus so much on nursing school that the attention you used to give to those closest to you will now appear nonexistent. The people you think would have supported you the most, now seem distant, and they may feel as if you are ignoring them. Maybe you are the only one in your family or group of friends of whom nursing is your calling. In this case, not only do you have a lack of support, but you don't have anyone else to talk to about it either. Some schools offer a therapist to their students due to the high amount of stress that comes with nursing school, but sometimes that just isn't enough. I know that I could recognize when I was stressed and had my share of mental disruptions during school. Truthfully, I did not want to spend even 30 minutes speaking to a therapist about it; I wanted more.

I wondered how beneficial it would be to have a mandatory universal course integrated into nursing programs across the world that focused on helping students recognize their heart condition and position. When I say condition, I mean have they been through so much that their hearts have grown cold or broken? Is their heart positioned where it is open not only to receiving but to giving love? Do they identify with the things they have gone through or are currently dealing with? People need to find their identity outside of what they are going to school for and learn the true wellness of their mind and heart. This is like prepping the soil and laying the foundation for people to be built up and flourish. Without these small beginnings, we will only have a "house" that will topple over when a small storm passes through. That's why it is so important for me to write this book for all of you. I really want to bring your focus toward the issue that begins within your heart. At the end of this book, I want to transform your way of looking at nursing as well as help you incorporate new techniques of compassion into your education and your nursing career. If we could correct our ways to follow the philosophy that compassion heals better than any medicine could, then we would have the ability to change the world of healthcare. Just imagine the millions of people that will be impacted with complete and whole healing. More and more nurses would finally feel whole and they would feel truly accomplished.

CHAPTER 2

Competence

I started my nursing journey in 2009. I was a senior in high school desperately searching for my purpose. I was ready to graduate and begin working toward my life long career goals. By the end of senior year, I realized that I hadn't been doing well academically, and I told myself that there was no way I'd get into the nursing program I wanted. I didn't feel like waiting a year or two before I was "considered" for a spot in a nursing program. I say "considered" because you don't just get accepted into a nursing program of your choice that easily. You will have to prove yourself through your previous academic history, provide references and get interviews. If a school doesn't like what they see on paper, your application may get "lost" under piles of others.

I always felt that if a school would just give me a chance at an interview, they could see my compassion for nursing and see that I was more than a perfect fit for their program. Unfortunately, many schools never gave me that opportunity and shut me down without a second thought. No matter what, I knew in my heart and soul that having an important role in health care was my childhood dream. I would remind myself that I could not allow someone else's opinion of my capabilities to stop me from pursuing my dreams. Through several attempts to hold my head up, I did let fear sink in and change my perception of who I was and what I was capable of doing. I reached for what I thought would be the easiest way to my dream job and I applied to a technical school to become a medical assistant. I figured that this path would allow me to gain knowledge and earn a degree faster than a traditional college which would then catapult me into the health care field.

That did not go as planned though, because life circumstances made it challenging for me to continue forward. I withdrew from the program in the second semester and decided that I wanted to be more than a medical assistant. More importantly, I felt like I was cheating my dreams and downplaying what I was called to do. I went to my local community college, still attempting to rush through a program. I craved any possible way to quickly jump into their nursing program. You'd think by now I would have learned that a fast track to becoming a nurse did not work before. Before I knew it, I changed programs two semesters in, and took classes that had nothing to do with my goals. I even remember completely walking away from campus without proper notice. As a result, my record showed an entire semester of failure. I let my personal issues get in the way, relationships distracted me, and excuses pile up. Once again, fear came knocking again and I opened the door. Do you see a pattern yet?

I snagged a job at my local nursing home, working as an activity aide so that I could at least be around people doing what I wanted to eventually do. As the weeks passed, every day became harder than the last. I knew in my heart I was meant to stand where those doctors and nurses stood. I worked at my job for nearly a year before I found out I was carrying my very first blessing. Yeah, you guessed it! I was pregnant. I used it as another excuse though, to eventually get me out of my job due to unhappiness.

I quit my job 7 months into my pregnancy, partly because I was exhausted and partly due to me feeling unaccomplished. I was lost in my identity of who I was and I got caught up watching everyone around me reach their goals. Scared and feeling of little worth, I left with more excuses to cover up the fact that I just was not happy with where I was at in my life. I taught myself how to do acrylic and gel nails, so I did that on the side to stay busy and maintain my sanity once my son was born. Once again, I found myself feeling like something was still missing.

One day while doing a friend's nails, I told her about my struggle of starting and stopping school, and how my real passion was in healthcare. She stopped me mid-sentence and immediately reached into her bag and pulled out a piece of paper. On it were instructions on how to get into a licensed practical nursing (LPN) program. She told me all about the program and encouraged me to apply with her so we could go to school with one another. She said there was still time to sign up and that she believed that I could do it. In that moment, a spark ignited within me that eventually turned into a fire that was burning for success. I did everything that I was supposed to do to get into the program. I purchased a study book for the TEAS entrance exam, which is an exam you need to pass to get into nursing programs. My friend and I studied together and took every mock test inside the practice book. Then the day came for my test. I was nervous the entire time. While taking the exam I thought to myself, "What in the world does this question even mean?!" Some of the material in the test was stuff from HIGH SCHOOL and it absolutely intimidated me because I barely remembered how to answer some of those questions. Although everything went well, I answered all the questions, not leaving and blank (even if I didn't know the answer). I still finished with fear following me.

It seemed like forever before they finally called me, about a week or so after the exam to say I was invited to a second interview (the first interview was prior to testing for a first impression). The date came, and I was interviewed by the program director. She discussed my test results with me and went over the areas I needed improvement on. Not even halfway through the interview, with a giant smile on her face, she was pleased to invite me into the LPN program. I can't explain how overwhelmed with joy I was at that moment. Most of her words after that sounded mumbled as I tried to wrap my mind around the fact that I was finally accepted into a nursing program. My dreams were finally coming true and I was determined with every single cell in my body to begin strong, continue strong, and finish even STRONGER. See, you can easily create a movie in your mind all from one negative thought and it can eventually tear you down mentally. I did that to myself over and over prior to LPN school and even afterwards. Now, I realize that you simply cannot worry about what tomorrow will bring. You can't focus on a negative thought because then you give it power to grow deep roots in your mind. Every time you begin to think negatively, you're just watering those roots and the "gloom tree" grows. In the outside, you may not even be experiencing those negative events, but on the inside, you created a monster of deception and fear. Uproot your "gloom tree," cast out all your fears and worries, and begin asking "what if something GOOD happens?"

So, nursing school began, and what I like to call "nursing school bliss" filled the air. You know, it's that feeling of heaven-sent excitement. You get all your medical books and syllabi and you are running on a full tank of perseverance. That bliss only lasted so long because challenges set in and school got REAL. Students started dropping out or failing out and our class size kept getting smaller and smaller as time went on. Scores of one hundred percent slowly dropped down to as low as fifty percent. Tests became harder and professors stopped handing out second chances. At the time, my son was an 8-month-old breastfed baby, so pumping became a part time job while attending school. With the responsibilities and challenges that I faced at home, I became weary, however, my spirit never allowed me to give up, even during what appeared to be the hardest time in my life.

It has taken me until now to see that within the midst of your weakness, you are building incredible strength for the next task God will assign to you in life. School was tough, and it made my personal life even tougher. I struggled, but I persisted. Even on the worst days with the little support I had, I told myself I was going to finish out strong. I knew that I would soon walk across a stage in short of 10 months with my diploma in my hand. There were days when I questioned whether I made the right choice, but there were even more days where I was sure that I was chosen for this path. I remembered how I started something only to turn around and quit too many times in the past, so this time it was not an option.

I went back to the times I prayed to get into nursing school and the day my prayer was answered. I thought about how many nights and days I spent praying for a breakthrough, for a change in my life, and finally reach the calling that I one hundred percent knew God had put in my life. I also remembered who was watching me. I wanted to be the best example for my little boy.

My entire class prepared for graduation with our speeches and dressed in white graduation caps and gowns. The moment they announced my name and read my speech, my eyes filled with tears. I sobbed the whole way up. I gave my instructors a hug as I received my diploma. It was as if time stood still and I could look at myself from the seats down below. I saw a woman who was broken several times. I saw someone who struggled consistently but now she stood tall, stronger than ever before. I could hardly look at any of my friends or family when I was on that stage. All the countless tears and sleepless nights finally paid off and the most important people in my life were able to witness it.

The feelings I had were so intense. It was an indescribable feeling of accomplishment that revealed to me that God was indeed with me. I got through school with a new baby and with the challenges of being a young mother. I had SO MANY opposing obstacles in my life, some days not knowing how I would even get to school. In those moments, I knew that God held me up the entire time. He had His hand over my life and I was blessed with support from every angle. For that, I am forever grateful.

After graduation, I immediately scheduled and studied for the NCLEX exam. Every day, I dedicated one hour to studying and within 3 weeks I was taking my test for licensure. I thought the TEAS exam was tough, but the NCLEX was on another level of hard. It was super challenging; however, I went in confidently knowing that I was competent enough to pass. During the exam, the computer shut off after 75 questions, which was the minimum number of questions one could answer. My heart sunk. I was told previously that many people believed that if you were shut off at 75 questions, then nine times out of ten you passed. On the contrary, my instructor also said sometimes the exam will shut off because you didn't do well at all. My gut was telling me I passed, and I thought to myself, there was no way I failed terribly. The questions were extremely tricky, but you know what? I finished. I was relieved to be done with tests and studying for hours on end. I could finally walk out of the testing facility and go home. Seriously, I felt like throwing my hands up and screaming. I got in my car and as I closed my eyes to cry, the only thing I could say was, "Thank you, God!"

You see, I knew I was never really alone, even during the moments when I felt alone. I knew He was the one that carried me through the challenging test during that season in my life. I knew He had given me relief, so I could rest knowing I did my best. So naturally, I did what all NCLEX test takers do, try the NCLEX "trick" to see if I passed. (Insert laughing emoji). It appeared to be a pass, but of course I had to wait one week before I received my actual results. Well, I finally received the official result of a PASS! What a weight lifted off my shoulders! I did it! And you know what? You can do it too. My story is a testimony for others to see that we have to overcome obstacles during periods of learning new things in order to reach the next level in life. Having challenges forces us to use the knowledge gained to move past those obstacles. Once we move past them, we can create a strategy to overcome the next challenge. This is knowledge that enables us, or better known as competency.

One of the main ingredients for "cooking up" the right nurse is competence. As a nurse, you will go through trials on your path to success. You will go through stages of suffering and sacrifice, crying and cheering, and laughter and enjoyment. Through it all, you will endure. Your education and the efforts you put in to truly absorb the information you are being taught, is a vital piece for you to be an amazing nurse. It's easy to feel overwhelmed with all the information you receive between clinicals and class hours, but it's essential that you really study. You must put in the time to comprehend the material. Don't allow fear stop you from asking questions. While you study, be prepared with at least 3 questions to ask your instructor for that next class. Meet with your instructor during their office hours. Schedule extra study time with your fellow classmates, and plan on giving your all to make sure you fully understand every lesson. Also, don't do it alone! Part of being successful is having a team. It takes a village to build. Don't remain stuck in thinking that it's all about you and you only. If everyone helps one another, the chances of all of you succeeding are much greater.

As a cake artist, I work on my own most, if not all of the time. I found that when I received help from friends and family, I am able to accomplish more in less time with little stress involved. I also reach out to other cake decorators or take part in seminars or videos so that I may become more competent in creating basic to complex cakes. Without the knowledge of baking and decorating, I wouldn't be able to sell, let alone create beautiful cakes. It takes time to study and a lot more time practicing in order to get better in my skills. I can't try to learn a whole bunch of material at once expecting to remember it all. I like to really study a skill and of course, without my support team backing me up and without other amazing cake artist guidance, I would not be able to be a successful cake artist.

One of the other key components to being a successful nurse is not to binge and purge the information you learn in nursing school. Sometimes I would think, "Do we really have to memorize and know ALL of this? Won't we have the internet and our drug guide right there to help?" Well, in my experience and opinion, yes. You really do need to memorize and know at least most of it. It not only benefits your future career working as a nurse, but if you want to continue your education (which I highly recommend), it will help you in so many ways.

You will soon go out into the world with the responsibility of being a valuable team member and the responsibility of healing many people. Strive to increase your knowledge, for your educational greatness! You can and will succeed! You are competent. You are capable. You are enough. Take the knowledge you acquired and never let it escape your mind. Your knowledge is something that NO ONE can take from you. Use it to propel you forward into the next journey you embark on. Most importantly, don't quit.

CHAPTER 3

Understanding

Sure, you may competently know something, but to have a true understanding is something different. I have countless examples from my personal experiences, so I will give a quick and simple one. Coming out of nursing school, pharmacology seemed almost permanently engraved in my brain. If you have taken the class already, you know what I am talking about. If you have not taken pharmacology yet or don't know what it is, let me briefly explain. Pharmacology is the study of medicine regarding the uses, effects, and actions of drugs. Going into the medical profession? You will have to take this class and be expected to learn, memorize, and pass lots of tests on what seems like an endless number of drugs.

When I began my first nursing job, I was prepared to give medications and I felt I was competent on what most drugs were. What I didn't realize is that I would soon have to learn how to literally explain these medications in terms that my patients would understand. For a while, my patients could tell that I was a brand-new nurse. I kept telling them, "I will double check for you and return with the answers to your questions."

How embarrassing! This is a great example of how you not only should "know" your stuff, but truly understand what you are doing as well as what you are working with. Knowing that a patient takes medications for pain and blood pressure is one thing, but you should be able to explain why they are taking it. It is key to tell them how it affects them positively and what possible negative side effects may occur. You can know the name of the medication and know that it is for pain relief, but you must also understand the medication and its function.

Another way misunderstanding can take place is skimming right past a patient you are assigned to care for when you're just trying to get the job done. If you ever worked in a facility where you oversee caring for 20 people or more, on most days you can see how skimming can come easily. I, personally, have worked as an LPN and visited several long-term/rehab care facilities where I have witnessed this. Everyone needs you and everyone needs something. Often, no matter where you work, being understaffed is common. Bells will go off, phones will ring non-stop, and physicians' orders will pile up. The people who you are assigned to care for, all rely on you day in and day out. In my experience of working, the nurse's workload is usually heavy and very demanding for just a single person. As a nurse, you are required to take care of people physically and also take care of people emotionally. Emotional care is crucial for a person's healing and well-being. If you are skimming through your day, you may miss meeting a patient's emotional needs. If I knew that I had one or more patients who needed extra emotional support, I would make a note of it and try to spend a little more time caring for them. It is so important to consider the point of view of your patient and see the situation from their eyes.

Understanding can come in many forms. You can understand someone in the sense that you clearly comprehend what they are saying, or you can understand someone in the sense that you are sympathetically aware of their feelings. The goal is to be able to clearly comprehend what someone is trying to express to you, whether verbal or non-verbal. However, it is also critically important that you carry the ability to be aware of your patient's feelings. Your level of care elevates to a higher standard when you can set aside your rushed way of thinking and feeling, to truly notice someone else's needs.

So many people in this world are misunderstood and it happens within the medical setting. Words get lost in translation between medical terminology or for example, if a nurse or doctor rushes through documentation, of which I have seen before. I would love to say I have seen nurses follow the rules of administering medications, but sadly I have seen the opposite. I have witnessed nurses not make themselves known to the patient and leave their medication on their bedside table. Some nurses ask their patients how they are doing. Some even take the time to briefly check the patient head to toe. But, for the most part, I've noticed that nurses make a quick stop in and then leave back out. It isn't to say they are a bad person or that they are purposely doing anything wrong, but can you see how quickly something can get missed? You might work in a facility where you see the same patients every single day like in long-term care, so you think you know them and their condition well enough. But in fact, they might be telling you something and it gets brushed off as a "behavior" or "mood" and it doesn't get fully understood.

Something I have learned to do is to take the time to truly understand where my patients are coming from. It can very well be a behavior or mood. They may complain about the same thing repeatedly to every nurse on every shift, but were you patient with them? Were you gentle and kind? Did you taken a couple extra minutes to empathize with them and let them know that you were aware of their feelings and wanted to help? I know it seems time consuming and right now you might be saying to yourself, "Is she nuts? Who has time for that?"

It makes a difference. You can't ever forget that you hold a title that is supposed to represent compassionate, healing care. You wear the title of healer and caretaker. So, in order to effectively understand your patients, you must take time to stop and actually listen to them. Listen to everything they say and how they say it. When you notice the beginning of apprehension or aggression, that is the perfect opportunity to show understanding, even if you are overwhelmed by their complaining. Try not to take anything personal and forgive them for any mean things they may have said in the midst of their anger. Make yourself aware of their true feelings. Ask why are they there to begin with? Are they alone? Do they have family? Does anyone come to visit them? Do they know that they are important and loved?

It is our duty as nurses to show them genuine understanding so that they can receive the best and highest quality of care. It is also important to allow the family members to be a part of the patient's healing. Sometimes I have seen nurses that don't take a moment to make the family aware that they are not alone in the journey of their loved one's healing. Let the family know that they are a part of the team and that we care about them as well. Through all the emotions and obstacles, let the family and the patient know you are walking through it with them too.

It kind of sounds funny throwing my comparison to cakes throughout this book, but it totally makes sense if you think about it. I understand how the ingredients work together to create the kind of cake I need for certain orders. Knowing how the ingredients work allows me to make a delicious cake for people who maybe are allergic to certain ingredients. For example, it's crucial to understand how eggs play an important part in baking a cake. If my client can't have eggs, then I am able to go ahead and substitute it with another ingredient that can function the same. Not only does my cake require understanding, but my customers need to be understood as well, just as my patients do. One time, I wasn't sure what my customer wanted as far as color arrangement on a cake. I tried to clarify via text messages on several occasions to get a better understanding on exactly what they had requested. However, I should have met with them in person or via phone call because I ended up misunderstanding and the order wasn't what they wanted. Therefore, understanding is not only key in nursing, but in all areas of life.

Just as you seek to be understood in your life, give the same to others. The beauty of it lies when all is said and done, when you genuinely understand the patient for who they are and what they are going through. People will begin to give you a gentle kindness in return. The next time you interact with someone, tuck away your feelings and really listen to what they are saying to you. No matter what they say or how they say it, try responding with kind words and a patient heart. You wouldn't believe the amount of joy that will fill your heart once you've spent a moment sharing kindness.

CHAPTER 4

Attention to Detail

How many of us are quick to glaze over a set of instructions, like taking on the project of building your tv stand, and it suddenly appears more difficult than you thought? The instructions that came with it have too many words and "A-B-C" parts, so you skip to the pictures to try to understand the directions better. You begin to build your project from the picture you are looking at and not from the actual worded instructions. You believe you have finally finished building your tv stand and then you realize the right-side paneling is inside out. At this point, everything has been put together, so in order to fix the paneling, you have to take everything apart. You say to yourself, "All of that hard work for nothing." Now, you don't even want to fix it, let alone have a tv stand at all. If only you had taken the time to pay attention to the details and maybe ask for help, you may have finished sooner. Instead you decided to skip over the details and rush to the end-product. All of that just to end up making a silly mistake and have to start from to the beginning. Do you get where I am going now?

One of the most important parts of being a successful student nurse and licensed/registered nurse, is paying attention to detail. I can't express how important it is for you to keep your mind focused when you are at work. It is crucial with every step you take while giving care. You could be administering medications or documenting in the patient's chart. It is too easy to get caught up in trying to get it all done quickly before lunch or before your shift is over. Carefully read the following scenarios I provided for some example scenarios.

Visualize being a new nurse and it's your first day on the job. You are super nervous and fail to realize that there were two patients with the same last name in the same exact room. You gave one patient the right medication but at the wrong time. You have now double dosed your patient on a pain medication. This happened so easily and so quickly, you didn't notice they had previously had it 2 hours ago. You definitely did not think something like this would ever happen to you. In another scenario, you are a seasoned nurse and you know these patients like the back of your hand. You've done this for years in many other jobs, but today you had an argument with your husband and you've been thinking about what he said. Your patient has a heart condition and you didn't check her apical pulse right before giving the medication like you were supposed to. Your mind is busy replaying the very hurtful words your husband said to you that morning which explains why you are "off your game". You give your patient the right medication but her parameters state to hold if her apical pulse is below 55 and her apical pulse was 49. She is a fragile cardiac patient, going into cardiac arrest and is rushed to the hospital. You have never done this before and usually her apical is always around 60, so you didn't think you needed to check it every single time.

When I bake a cake, everything can go wrong if I don't pay attention and it doesn't stop there. When I prep my cakes to stack or carve them, if I am distracted or trying to rush, I can completely ruin a whole order. Every single step of cake baking/decorating requires close attention to details. I really have to focus and get in the zone with minimal distractions to complete each edible masterpiece. The same awareness must go into nursing, because the way something detrimental can happen to one of my cakes, something detrimental can also happen to a patient.

I can't stress how important it is when you are dealing with a life. It could be the simplest thing that absolutely changes someone's day or changes their life forever. I know you want to be that compassionate nurse who stands above the rest. Focus on taking extra care when you are on the job. Some days it will be extremely tough to muster through with all the issues you have going on outside those work doors. But, when you oversee the well-being of others, your desire for your own good must shift to the desire for the good of others too. You will make some mistakes, it happens. I have had my fair share of mistakes too like the very first scenario. Thankfully none of them were detrimental.

It goes to show that no one is perfect. There is no perfect nurse or doctor in the world; every one of them have made a mistake at one point in their career, either a small silly one or on a larger scale. We can't control the actions of others, however, we do have the power to control our own, so be sure you always pay close attention, no matter the situation.

CHAPTER 5

Endurance

The ability to tolerate a difficult situation is what builds the character we need to excel in every aspect of life. Without this endurance, we tend to find ourselves in situations where we feel stuck. We begin to feel depleted or even withdrawn from what used to be our passion. All these feelings can manifest within you. They manipulate your mind until finally you literally see yourself broken down into pieces, no longer want to take another step into the nursing field again. However, if you are reading this, you probably have an interest in pursuing nursing, therefore you have it in you to thrive. Within a great nurse rests a person who perseveres. Never forget to remind yourself of your character so that it strengthens your perseverance. Take care of your health, as a whole, to build and maintain your physical and mental strength. If you want to truly heal others, you must remember that your well-being is also top priority.

We can't possibly expect to give the best care to others if our mind and body are not well. Take care of yourself. Fill your mind with positivity and goodness. Listen to soothing music that has purpose and brings you joy. Watch things that educate and empower your mind. I personally read the word of God to strengthen, encourage, and inspire me! The book of Psalm is SO powerful for this. Or, read books and articles that uplift. You can even reach out for counseling from a therapist or seek wise counsel from your pastor. Don't be afraid to ask for help. It takes a village, remember?

Talk to someone you can trust to safely express your feelings. Remove yourself from conversations that are pointless or filled with complaining and gossip. Fill your body with purifying and strengthening foods like fresh fruits and vegetables. Decrease or eliminate your consumption of processed sugars and foods that fog your mind and make you feel sluggish. It is amazing how energized a balanced meal can make you feel as opposed to a processed fast food meal. There is no price tag on life, and you are worthy of living happy and healthy.

Although creating cakes is my way of releasing stress and having fun, it can also bring on the stress with some of the cakes I customize. There have been plenty of times I would have one or more cake orders for some crazy cool cakes. When those kinds of orders come in, I can work on them for hours on end until I feel my cake artwork is complete. Often, I would be working on a cake for hours straight, not eating and forgetting to rehydrate myself. Then, I wouldn't get to bed until 4 in the morning and sometimes I wouldn't even sleep! I would work through the night into the morning, shower and take a nap until my customer came to pick up their order. This is totally unhealthy and soon I became extremely run down. I had zero endurance because I would not take care of my health which in turn caused other issues. Endurance is needed for anything you put your all into, including any other careers and even relationships.

When we build up mental and physical endurance from the inside, we can power through the most challenging times. It doesn't mean you won't cry or that you will be free from troubled days. It means that you will have the necessary strength to get back up after you have fallen so you can finish what you started. You decided to become a nurse for a reason (and hopefully it wasn't just to make a certain amount of money), to take part in the process of healing people wholly, from start to finish. You have it in you already. Remember, step one to building it up is caring for yourself entirely, starting from the inside.

CHAPTER 6

Honesty

Honesty is the key to building long lasting relationships and great rapport. Being honest is such a simple act. To be honest is to be completely real without any question of genuineness. If you aren't honest with anyone or with yourself, how will you maintain success? How will you ever be trusted with the greater things in life if you can't be trusted with the simpler things in life, like honesty? Living a lie on a day to day basis or partially walking in sincerity with no moral principles only sets you up for a life time of stress. You never reach true happiness or fulfillment by walking in the shadows and not being the REAL YOU. The stress of covering up the truth will eventually lead you into failure. When you carry yourself in the light of good character, you prepare yourself to receive great things in abundance.

It feels good to know that you have nothing to hide and that you work for what is right. When you live by the standard of true integrity, even if someone tries to make you feel wrong, no one can break you down. All your work in life up until now has been the basis for the construction of a sturdy "home" on a solid foundation. How have you been working in your life? Is your foundation weak? Will a single blow of the wind knock your house down? Integrity is a big part of having that solid foundation.

As nurses, if we do not hold ourselves accountable for our honesty, we can cause damage to others. If you see that something isn't being done correctly regarding care of a patient, are you that person that says, "Well, that isn't my patient, that nurse has to deal with that," or "I don't want to get involved, it's not my problem."? Do you think to yourself, "Well, it isn't that serious, they'll be okay."?

I have noticed some of the health care industry making changes to ensure that integrity is top priority. Some places state integrity is a part of their core values, but then some employees do not reflect that, as I have previously witnessed. I watched doctors not go in a patient's room but ask the nurse how the patient has been and then write it off as if they have checked on the patient themselves. There has been a time where I have seen a doctor prescribe a new medication they don't know much about or that they don't even fully believe in. The money appears to be top priority within healthcare. I also have seen doctors in such a hurry that they don't focus on how it will affect the patient. I have been the nurse to receive an order like that and question why that medication or why that dosage was chosen. I was taught to always get clarification if you are unsure about something. However, there were times the doctors have made me feel as if I did not know what I was talking about and ignore my concerns. Where does the integrity stand? The moral principle of a life being precious, no matter who it is, appears to have been forgotten these days. Every single person deserves an equal amount of honesty and to be treated with fairness.

I will never fail to make sure I properly educate my patients on whatever I do and on the care I provide them with. It can be as simple as telling them the truth about what they are taking and why it has been prescribed to them. I always made it a point to reassure them on their right to know as well as the right to refuse until further understanding is achieved. You must make your patient feel comforted and secure. You can't make someone feel like they can trust you if you are not being honest with them. Successful outcomes in patient care require honor and trust. When you give people an unscripted version of you, then you gain trust. You don't have to put on an act but you also must keep the professionalism.

It is amazing how many problems can be resolved when the trust is mutual. There is no need to try to be like someone else or to conform yourself into what you think a good nurse is made of. You became a nurse because it is already in you. You were already prequalified before you entered this field. You don't have to think hard to be a good nurse if you remember to remain honest and be yourself. Don't let anything distract you from holding onto your integrity. Unfortunately, there will be days where your integrity is tested. You might unfortunately witness nurses lying right before your eyes, or team members covering up for others. It's at that time where you have to make the decision to accept what you see and go along with everyone else, or boldly stand up for what is true.

I wish I had someone tell me this when I began working as a nurse. Honesty is key right? Well here is my time to share that I wasn't always 100% honest. I had trouble "fitting in" with other nurses, and truthfully, I had a lot of fear of negative confrontation, retaliation from co-workers, or possibly loss of my job. I did my best to hold on to my integrity but I watched it fall piece by piece as the weeks passed by. I got caught up in blending in and trying to not cause any problems with others at my job. Then it came to me. I hope you realize that you are one of a kind and were not made to blend in, especially if it costs you your integrity.

I eventually grew to a point where I gained courage and boldness at my job and did not care what anyone thought or said about me. I was not there to heal employees, I was there to heal my residents and give them the proper, honest care they needed. From that day forward, no fear stood in between that. As I built up my integrity, I realized I didn't ever have to try to keep it, because it is a part of me.

As a cake artist, honesty and integrity are also key components. A customer may come to you asking for this extravagant custom cake idea that you know you do not have the skills or maybe time to make it. You then need to be honest with yourself and with them to explain why you cannot take their cake order. If you end up taking the order and don't deliver their requests, you not only lose trust from that customer, but also future potential customers.

Sometimes the pressure of success can make us say and do things we probably shouldn't, like being dishonest. Do not let pressure or fear break down your integrity! Stand up for what's right and always be of good character.

CHAPTER 7

No Judgement

Some call them the drug seeker, the complainer, the racist, the hater, the gay one, or the he-she not sure what gender one. People are so quick to look at someone and instantly form an idea of what kind of person they are. In nursing, I watched it happen in every single place I have ever worked. Nurses have given me a report on a whole set of people I never had the opportunity to care for and "warn me." I know this isn't new to you if you've worked in the healthcare field already; you know exactly what I am talking about. "Oh this guy complains of pain every 30 minutes. He's is a drug seeker so be careful. This other patient takes advantage of you and will cry out all day, just don't pay them any mind because they do it all the time."

I wonder why then not try and help these people overcome? These patients, no matter what kind of healthcare setting they are in, are bound to the hospital or whatever facility they are in, and they're most likely confined to a bed or wheelchair. They might be dealing with a list of problems that need real solutions, not maintenance.

You didn't earn your title to choose who you want and who you don't want to give the best care to. You didn't work your butt off in school and sacrifice so much to work and not make a difference for those you are giving care to. It may seem like you are the only one who is trying, but your efforts make a bigger impact than you think. If you only ever help one person overcome, you have changed a WHOLE life. You don't know if that person will go on to be the greatest writer of all time, or if they will go on to become a doctor and heal many lives themselves. You have no idea if one day, you become ill and the aide or nurse taking care of you was that same person you failed to give proper care based on your judgement.

Respect is key. We are not the judge of who deserves a certain amount of respect. Every single living thing deserves the same amount of respect. One person is not worthier than the another. It is sad to see lack of respect to other team members. I have seen nursing aides that constantly pick up after the last shift's half executed work. I have also come across housekeepers that stay late to make sure the rooms are sparkling clean and disinfected but receive little respect. In a career of caring, you will have to serve others no matter what shape, color, or size. You have a responsibility to be a part of the healing process regardless of how you identify with people.

The identity of a person does not lie in opinions; it doesn't lie in their mistakes or their past. Treat your patients and all members of the team with respect. Be polite and let positivity radiate from you. Begin to look at everyone as a whole and not just one piece of them. Listen to what they have to say about their own life and experiences. Take a moment to find out a little more about them as an individual. Find out from their medical records (if you are authorized) or from family and friends what it is that the patient used to do or what they like to do now. Do they like music? Were they an artist? Do they have children or grandchildren that bring them joy when they come to visit?

Provide your patients with judgement-free comfort. Let them know that you are there for their healing and care, not to judge their character based on their condition or their past. Communicate with your staff and don't go into work with that saying, "I am not here to make friends, I am here to work." Of course, you are there to work, but everyone works better together if treated like a team or a big family. So get to know one another and don't pose judgement on them. Come to work saying, "I am here to encourage and uplift my team. I am a vital part of the staff. I am ready to make a difference." I understand not every day will be this way. I have had days where I felt like I was completely over it, especially when some co-workers managed to make me feel out of place. I also know it's tough to deal with a person or a group of people who give off an attitude or are always rude.

When I am handling my cake customers, I am always sure to be

100 percent honest with them about pricing and what they will be receiving. I have seen other cake bakers that will not want to spend much time with a potential customer because they don't look like they can afford it. I try to make every single customer feel just as special as the next. I take my time with each customer, assuring they feel comfortable with every step of the ordering process. I also learned to ask plenty of questions and allow my customers to ask questions so that we both achieve full understanding of their order. Despite all of this, even in the cake business I ran into trouble with customers who have been upset and dissatisfied. I experienced customers who were very rude and although I did my best to come to a solution for them, they still managed to share an attitude towards me.

But, did you know you can be the place where that attitude ends? When you respond with negativity, it spreads faster than the flu. I've found a great response to be, "I understand you are upset, and it's okay. I am here to be the solution and not the continuation of a problem. What can I do to help?" It is hard for someone to come back at you with more negativity with that kind of reply.

It does not matter what color, size, shape, illness, or gender someone is. Everyone is going through life all at different paces and in different stages, but not one single person deserves less care and love than the next. Give respect and be a place of comfort. Healing will begin to take place instead of brokenness, within yourself and within others.

CHAPTER 8

Compassion

Oh compassion. We finally reach the main ingredient, and possibly the most important ingredient, to be a great nurse. Like baking a cake, you can't skip any ingredient or it just won't taste right. But, if you miss the main ingredient, you won't even bake anything that looks like a cake. The same goes for nursing, you just won't get a good nurse without that aspect of caring!

When you go to nursing school, they teach you all the technical things you need to know to prepare you for your career as a nurse. Your instructors might briefly skim over compassion (with emphasis on might). I think the amount of material we need to learn and study, creates no room to spend on talking about the importance of compassion. I attended a school where we spent an hour or so learning about the mental/emotional aspect of nursing, but we did not really discuss compassion. We all know that nursing is a caring profession. However, I think it easily gets boxed up and labeled as the knowledge of physically caring for someone. Sure, you can be the best at physically caring for someone, but with what emotion are you providing care?

Here is where position of heart comes into play. Another key is having a willing and caring heart. Nursing isn't for those who are solely looking for a certain salary, or at least it shouldn't be. Nursing also isn't for those who are seeking a title to prove something. It also isn't for those who think they can choose which patients they will and won't care for. Unfortunately, the nursing field has a good mix of nurses like this. People chasing "the bag" and concerned with having a set of two or three letters after their name. It is truly unfair to those that desire to really be a healer of many, giving every ounce of their heart and soul into caring.

This profession requires you to no longer put yourself as the main concern. Instead, your patients' well-being is your top priority. You will walk into work and what ever you have going on in your life will have to stay outside those doors. I know many of you have probably heard this at school or work, but it's true. You just can't wear your problems on your face and body when you go to care for someone's life. Think about a baby - would you want someone who came to work at your baby's daycare have a sense of aggression or attitude? Absolutely not! So, what makes it any different at your job? You will get tired and you might feel like throwing your whole nursing title in the trash some days, but you must remain compassionate.

Compassion is what pushes me through my worst days, believe it or not. Compassion is also what propels me through my best days. When I provide care to anyone, I look at it as an opportunity given to me to bring that sick or hurt person closer to their health and wellness goals. I take the time to look at my patient in the eyes and smile, asking if there is anything I can do that day to make their day easier. I do my best to be gentle when I speak. I am slow to anger when I am approached with negativity. I also always let them know that I am there to serve them and assist in their healing journey. This kind of compassion allows your patient to feel warmth from your caring heart. Your patient will then feel comfort with your presence.

A lot of nurses don't necessarily care to humble themselves and see eye-level with their patients or other staff members. It shouldn't have to take a family member visiting, or the state survey agency coming to your facility for you to clothe yourself in compassion. It is amazing how many amazing staff members and caring nurses you will see when "state" is coming. It shouldn't have to take the state surveyors to come to finally see things in order. When I decorate a cakes in fondant, if my cake has a hole on the side, no amount of icing will stop that hole from showing through the fondant. The same goes for compassion. You can't temporarily act compassionate to cover up the lack thereof. This is not something you think about; it is just something you carry. It's present when you love what you do. My cake customers can see the care and love I put into every order. Your compassion shows and speaks for itself in your work, whatever it may be.

Tough days won't cease, so value each day you have to make a positive impact on this earth. You have come too far to give up now. The beauty that lives within you was meant to shine and be a guide for others. Carry peace in your mind and share it with those around you. Focus also on valuing the life you are caring for, because after all, you have the power to make a positive or negative impact on them. Healthcare team members must join and strive for better. Compassion cannot be bought. Successful healthcare businesses, companies, and facilities must pour compassion over their employees so that it can overflow onto the millions in need of care. Compassion doesn't start at the problem. It should be the primary ingredient for the foundation of which health care stands on. Some solutions may be to hire more nurses, aides, cooks, environmental safety, and maintenance to create larger teams for each shift. Time must be taken to give all members of the healthcare team equal special attention for training. Human beings are not a number on a ticket dispensed from a machine. I've also noticed a lot of places will not hire LPNs with little or no experience whether in the field they're hiring in or in general. Everyone has to start somewhere, experience is gained. Maybe it's time for employers to hire the less experienced who are highly motivated and compassionate. With proper training and a chance, they can then receive the experience they need.

    A suggested solution for health care facility owners would be to come in and check on their employees and business more often. Doing this will allow them to see what can be added to create and maintain a more positive environment. New in-services and educational trainings can be created to will empower and motivate the entire team to want to serve better. Nursing care teams can be strengthened by acknowledging of those who put their all into what they do there. Support needs compassion, and without compassion, whole healing can't begin. The entire healthcare team requires equal support from one another. No one is beneath another just because one holds a higher title.

Without compassionate support, motivation is lost. Stress increases and it leaks into every part of the interdisciplinary team. Not only do we suffer, but the patients suffer. Our co-workers are not only our team, but our healthcare "family." Everyone should really provide good intentional care to their teams for them to overcome challenges and achieve success. Support can be expressed by sharing motivating words, focusing and magnifying the positives in each individual instead of picking at their flaws. Support can be given by valuing every person and the work they do. Through my own personal experience and asking several nurses of all kinds, I found that many nurses feel undervalued, underappreciated and undercompensated. All of which are things that can be improved when we begin to also have compassion for the members of the health care team. I've seen that when nurses feel important and feel cared about, the quality of care provided improves significantly.

Compassion heals. It allows for a step towards success. It rains positivity and love, truly making a difference in care. A lot of the world is missing out on this very important "ingredient" of compassion and this is the reason I was led to write this book. The goal of the book is to help "cook-up" some amazing nurses. These nurses will create foster creativity for innovative solutions. They will lead extraordinary successful teams. Nurses and student nurses: you are essential and you chose a beautiful career. The world so desperately needs compassionate nurse leaders. Let's come together to build each other up stronger.

You can be the "cure" to the problem in health care, but it starts with your heart. With the correct positioning of your heart, you can successfully lead with compassion at the forefront. Where is your heart positioned? Are you prepared to deal with extremely difficult cases of people in need of healing? Be willing to put aside your desire to get home on time and stay a few more minutes and make sure your job is fully done.

Be competent, ask questions and stay informed. Be understanding while giving respect. Carefully listen to others, showing empathy. Be attentive to little details just as much as the big ones. Be aware of not only what is best for you, but what is best for the patient. Take care of yourself to avoid being "burnt out." Power through the tough days and use them to strengthen you to strive for greatness. Be honest. Don't cut corners. Hold on to your integrity and be you.

Do your best to be non-judgmental. People, whether broken or whole, are still a valuable life with purpose. Show kindness and give support to one another. Magnify the positives in one another especially in stressful situations. And finally, be the compassionate nurse.

In the back of this book I have attached two nursing help sheets that I have created for you to use to your advantage. The first one is called a "nursing cheat sheet." It was created to assist nursing students and nurses quickly prioritize and organize important tasks for their shift. I created it for myself while working in the rehabilitation/long-term care setting, because it became increasingly stressful and difficult to try and keep track of certain important tasks. The second sheet is a detailed nursing report for patients who are on your 24-hour report. It gives you a bigger picture on an individual patient. I like to use this sheet also for everyone I will be assigned to care for during my shift. You can come in earlier and obtain this information for your shift or have your nursing facility implement these to make it easier for nurses to complete charting and report off with.

DATE: _____   ASSIGNED ROOMS: _____

NURSING REPORT

CNAs :   Other Nurses:

24 Hour Charting   LABS/ETC.

Glucose Checks

Treatments   IVs

1200 Meds   1400 Meds

DETAILED SHIFT REPORT   Date:

Name & Age	FULL / DNR / DNI / Other:
Rm #	Meds: CRUSH WHOLE Diet
Doctor	Appointments
Allergies	Therapy
Dx	
Mental Status	Functional Status
O2 L via % sat	Labs	Urine/BM

IV Site:	Date:	Drsg Change:
ABT	Isolation	Skin Condition

Glucose Checks

0630	1130	1630	2100

Vital Signs

BP: /   T: P: R:

Status Changes During Shift:

ABOUT THE AUTHOR

Living in sunny Florida, Luzmarie "Luma" Hawkins is a jack of all trades. She is known for her different self-taught talents in art especially with cakes. She has competed in Florida's SoFlo Cake & Candy Expo Miami in 2018 as well as showcased her edible masterpieces in several art shows in upstate NY. She grew up a U-E Tiger from Endicott, NY and went on to obtain her diploma in nursing. She is also known for her compassion specifically as a licensed practical nurse of five years among long-term care, rehabilitation facilities, home health care, women's health and integrative medicine. She has volunteered in The Great Teach-In where she educated elementary students on being both a cake artist and a nurse. She has a profound love for Christ, gaining more knowledge and wisdom about the word of God every day. Inspiration and encouragement have been key in her life as she hopes to share it with millions through her writing and her blog *Luma's Layers.*

www.ingramcontent.com/pod-product-compliance
Lightning Source LLC
Chambersburg PA
CBHW051334220526
45468CB00004B/1640